NUTRITION FOR BRAIN HEALTH

Fighting Dementia

Laura Town and
Karen Kassel

Ω
OMEGA
PRESS

Ω Omega Press
Zionsville, IN

Production Credits:
Authors: Laura Town and Karen Kassel
Editor: Amanda Boyle
Publisher: Omega Press
Photos: All images used under license from Shutterstock.com

ISBN 10: 0-9969832-2 -8
ISBN 13: 978-0-9969832-8

Social media connections:
Laura Town
Twitter: @laurawtown

Karen Kassel
Twitter: @KarenKassel1

NUTRITION FOR BRAIN HEALTH: FIGHTING DEMENTIA

Dementia is a term used to describe a group of symptoms, including memory loss, decline in social abilities, and changes in thinking patterns. The most common form of dementia is Alzheimer's disease, which makes up approximately 60 to 80 percent of all dementia cases. Currently, no absolute prevention or cure exists for dementia, but individuals can make changes to their daily dietary and exercise habits to help reduce their risk of developing dementia.

Recent research suggests that specific dietary changes can help increase memory. These nutritional guidelines can benefit both those who wish to decrease their risk of developing dementia and those hoping to slow the progression of the disease. Similarly, some dietary changes are specific either for preventative means or to delay the progression of the disease.

Decreasing Risk Factors

Individuals with multiple risk factors for developing dementia, including Alzheimer's disease, should consider making several nutritional changes. Many of these changes are easy to incorporate into daily dietary habits, such as increasing daily consumption of coffee to three to five cups, drinking a cup or two of green or black tea, and eating more fruits and vegetables. Other changes are more intensive, depending on your current diet, including ensuring a healthy and balanced diet and participating in a regular exercise routine.

Research has shown that certain additions to a person's diet can dramatically decrease the chance of developing dementia, or at the very least slow onset of the disease by years. These changes work to improve both body and brain health. Because being overweight in middle adulthood can increase the risk of developing dementia, some of the same dietary modifications that improve body and brain health can help decrease obesity, which in turn helps prevent the development of dementia.

Nutrition and Obesity

A healthy body mass index may lower the risk of developing dementia, especially Alzheimer's disease. Body mass indexes within the overweight and obese ranges correlate with Alzheimer's disease diagnoses later in life. Therefore, maintaining balanced nutrition and participating in regular exercise throughout life are vitally important. In addition, healthy food choices involving less saturated fats, as well as choosing foods responsible for lowering cholesterol, can be very helpful in preventing or delaying the onset of dementia. Lowering cholesterol and decreasing saturated fat intake can also help improve your health overall and decrease your risk factors for heart disease and stroke.

Adult BMI Chart

BMI	19	20	21	22	23	24	25	26	27	28	29	30	31	32	33	34	35
Height	Weight in Pounds																
4'10"	91	96	100	105	110	115	119	124	129	134	138	143	148	153	158	162	167
4'11"	94	99	104	109	114	119	124	128	133	138	143	148	153	158	163	168	173
5'	97	102	107	112	118	123	128	133	138	143	148	153	158	163	168	174	179
5'1"	100	106	111	116	122	127	132	137	143	148	153	158	164	169	174	180	185
5'2"	104	109	115	120	126	131	136	142	147	153	158	164	169	175	180	186	191
5'3"	107	113	118	124	130	135	141	146	152	158	163	169	175	180	186	191	197
5'4"	110	116	122	128	134	140	145	151	157	163	169	175	180	186	192	197	204
5'5"	114	120	123	132	138	144	150	156	162	168	174	180	186	192	198	204	210
5'6"	118	124	130	136	142	148	155	161	167	173	179	186	192	198	204	210	216
5'7"	121	127	134	140	146	153	159	166	172	178	185	191	198	204	211	217	223
5'8"	125	131	138	144	151	158	164	171	177	184	190	197	203	210	216	223	230
5'9"	128	135	142	149	155	162	169	176	182	189	196	203	209	216	223	230	236
5'10"	132	139	146	153	160	167	174	181	188	195	202	209	216	222	229	236	243
5'11"	136	143	150	157	165	172	179	186	193	200	208	215	222	229	236	243	250
6'	140	147	154	162	169	177	184	191	199	206	213	221	228	235	242	250	258
6'1"	144	151	159	166	174	182	189	197	204	212	219	227	235	242	250	257	265
6'2"	148	155	163	171	179	186	194	202	210	218	225	233	241	249	256	264	272
6'3"	152	160	168	176	184	192	200	208	216	224	232	240	248	256	264	272	279
	Healthy Weight						Overweight					Obese					

Credit: U.S. Department of Health and Human Services

Decrease saturated fats and cholesterol

Most people have heard of saturated fats and cholesterol, both of which are generally perceived to be negative components of a diet. However, both of these are important parts of a person's daily dietary nutrition when consumed in moderation. Saturated fatty acids are the "solid fats" found in many animal-based foods, such as butter, cream, fatty meats, and cheese. Consuming some of these foods is not bad; the negative health risks arise when you eat too much food containing saturated fats. Unsaturated fats are considered to be healthier for a person than saturated fats, because they can help improve blood cholesterol levels and are not as likely to lead to weight gain. Unsaturated fatty acids can be found in many plant-based foods, as well as some oils, such as olive oil, peanut oil, and corn oil. However, although unsaturated fats are healthier than saturated fats, they should still be eaten in moderation.

A high intake of saturated fatty acids leads to an increase in cholesterol. Two types of cholesterol exist: HDL (high density lipoprotein) cholesterol ("good" cholesterol) and LDL (low density lipoprotein) cholesterol ("bad" cholesterol). Bad cholesterol leads to the formation of thick, hard plaques that accumulate in a person's arteries, making them inflexible. Inflexible or blocked arteries can inhibit blood flow and increase the risk of developing heart disease. In addition, high levels of bad cholesterol are associated with an increased risk of developing dementia, including Alzheimer's disease. This correlation is hypothesized to be due to several factors, such as decreasing the efficiency of blood flow to the heart, which also decreases blood flow to the brain. If the brain is not receiving enough oxygen-rich blood, then its functionality will decrease and damage can occur, which could speed the development of plaques and tangles in the brain, leading to Alzheimer's disease.

Foods that contain saturated fatty acids include both meat and dairy products. Meat products that are high in saturated fats usually involve fat from the meat itself; for example, fatty beef, pork, and lamb are all high in saturated fat, as is the skin from poultry. Saturated fats are also found in dairy products such as butter, lard, cream, and some types of cheeses. Having some saturated fats in your diet is fine; the problem arises when an excess of them are consumed daily. As long as 5% to 6% or less of your daily caloric intake comes from saturated fats, the amount is not seen as dangerous in most cases. However, if 15% of your daily intake is made up of saturated fats, you are at risk for high cholesterol and thus at an increased risk for Alzheimer's disease and dementia.

Many foods that are high in saturated fats are also high in calories. This essentially means that not only can these foods contribute to high cholesterol, they can also lead to weight gain. Maintaining a healthy weight is imperative to decreasing your risk for dementia. Individuals with higher body mass indexes have a greater likelihood of developing dementia later in life when compared to those with lower body mass indexes. This is likely due to the fact that lower calorie consumption aids in protective brain chemical processes, which help the brain in recovering from injuries or degenerations such as Alzheimer's disease. One way to decrease saturated fat intake and maintain a healthy body weight is to focus on consuming a healthy, balanced diet.

Healthy balanced diet

A healthy and balanced diet is an important factor to consider when working to prevent Alzheimer's disease or dementia. Having a poor diet containing too much of one type of food and not enough of another can damage your brain. This is especially true if you are consuming too much sugar or saturated fat on a daily basis. The best defense, in terms of food and beverage consumption, is to ensure that your diet is both healthy and balanced. This does not mean that you have to give up high-sugar foods all together, but rather that they should be eaten in moderation and in conjunction with other healthy food options.

In order to have a balanced diet, you should have a daily mix of whole grains, grains, protein, fruits, vegetables, dairy products, and different types of oils. Each of these food groups should be consumed every day in different amounts, but because they are such broad groups you still have a lot of options. The following checklist discusses some tips for consuming a balanced diet with essential nutrients.

Checklist: Tips for a balanced diet

- **Grains.** Daily grain consumption should be an even mix between refined grains and whole grains. If your daily recommended grain consumption is 6 ounces, then 3 of those ounces should be whole grains, such as whole wheat pasta, brown rice, or buckwheat products.

- **Protein.** Daily protein consumption can be satisfied with several different types of foods, including lean meats, eggs, beans, fish, seafood, soy products, and nuts and seeds.
- **Fruits.** A variety of fruit types should be consumed to get the most nutrients. Raw fruits generally have more nutritional value than store-bought fruit juices.
- **Vegetables.** When choosing vegetables, they should be a mix of red, orange, green, and starchy vegetables.
- **Dairy.** Dairy products can include milk, cheese, yogurt, ice cream, and sour cream. Low-fat or fat-free dairy products are healthier than dairy products containing fat, because much of the fat in dairy products is saturated fat. In addition, the calcium contained in dairy products is more readily absorbed in the presence of vitamin D.
- **Oils.** Oils, while not a food group, are an important part of a healthy diet because they provide essential nutrients. Olive oil is a healthier oil to cook with than vegetable oil or butter. Solid fats, such as lard, butter, and bacon grease, are much less healthy to cook with than the majority of oils.

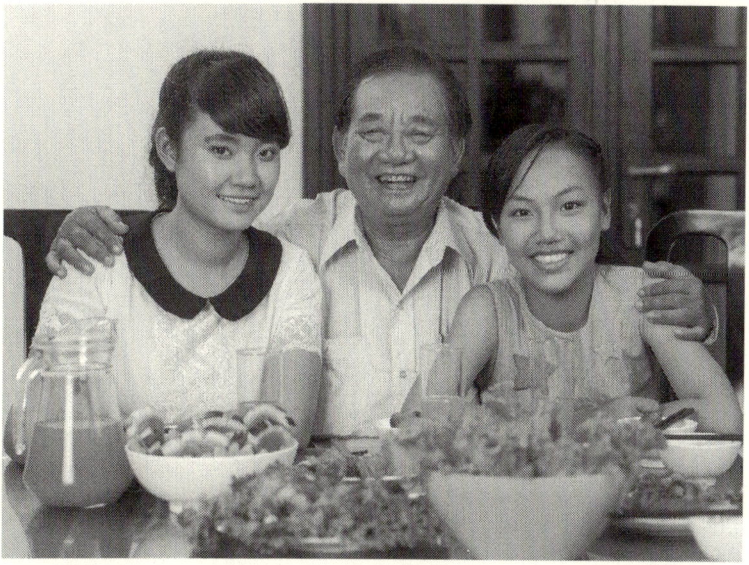

Credit: Dragon Images

The nutritional information included on most food products is based on a 2,000 calorie a day diet, but this is not always the healthiest option for all individuals. For example, those who are not very physically active during the day, getting less than 30 minutes of exercise, may only need 1,600 or 1,800 calories a day. Women, in particular, generally need fewer calories a day than men. While some people may need less than 2,000 a day to maintain a healthy weight or lose excess weight, others may need 2,400 or even 2,600 calories a day to prevent abnormal weight loss. This is generally true of individuals who are active more than 60 minutes a day and currently have a healthy weight range or individuals who have a metabolic disorder that causes unwanted weight loss. One way to determine how many calories you should consume each day would be to check an online food plan generator, such as the one at Choose MyPlate, a government resource sponsored by the USDA. Generators such as this one will ask your current weight, height, age, and activity level and then suggest a healthy calorie range based on these factors. Those with health concerns or special dietary needs should consult their doctors about any changes in their regular dietary habits. The following checklist provides the suggested daily amounts for each food group based on different calorie requirements.

Checklist: Daily Nutrition

1,600 Calorie Diet

- Grains: 5 ounces
- Fruit: 1 ½ cups
- Vegetables: 2 cups
- Dairy: 2 ½ cups
- Protein: 5 ounces

1,800 Calorie Diet

- Grains: 6 ounces
- Fruit: 1 ½ cups
- Vegetables: 2 ½ cups
- Dairy: 3 cups
- Protein: 5 ounces

2,000 Calorie Diet

- Grains: 6 ounces
- Fruit: 2 cups
- Vegetables: 2 ½ cups
- Dairy: 3 cups
- Protein: 5 ½ ounces

2,200 Calorie Diet

- Grains: 7 ounces
- Fruit: 2 cups
- Vegetables: 3 cups
- Dairy: 3 cups
- Protein: 6 ounces

Portion size is very important when considering a balanced diet. Many people do not realize how small portion sizes should be to adhere to the calorie requirements for a 2,000 calorie or less diet. For example, a hamburger that contains a quarter pound of meat—the typical size of a small hamburger—is four ounces of protein. For a 2,000 calorie a day diet, that one hamburger makes up almost your entire allotment of protein for the day. The amount of food that is served at restaurants is often much greater than the recommended daily amounts as well. Consider a typical steak dinner at a restaurant. Normally, steaks served at restaurants are between 6 and 12 ounces and come with sides ranging from potatoes and cooked vegetables to a serving of French fries. If you eat the whole steak, you could actually consume up to twice the amount of protein recommended for the day and a large portion of saturated fat as well. If a baked potato is served with the meal, that is approximately 1 cup or more from your vegetable requirement for the day, and if you add butter and sour cream to your potato, you are again increasing saturated fat consumption. If you also have cooked vegetables on the side, you could get close to 2 cups of vegetables in one meal. All of this is not even including any appetizers, bread, or dessert that was served with the meal. Many restaurants are now required to have calorie counts listed on the menu, so portions are a bit easier to estimate, but it is still good practice to consider how much is being consumed when working to achieve a balanced diet.

By consuming a balanced diet, in place of having all protein and no vegetables or all grains and no protein, it allows your body to function at optimal health. Operating at optimal health essentially means that your whole body benefits—including your brain. One common misconception is that the food you eat does not impact your brain health, and thus does not contribute to Alzheimer's disease or dementia. In reality, the food an individual consumes has a direct impact on brain functionality. Foods that are high in sugar or fat slow down brain activity, because they eventually lead to high insulin levels. When the high insulin levels begin to recede, a "sugar crash" occurs, in which you begin to feel sluggish, tired, and unable to process information as quickly as before. If these "crashes" occur frequently, they can cause physical, lasting damage to the memory centers of your brain.

Consuming a balanced diet helps eliminate chances for further damage by supplying the brain with nutrients needed to function at optimal capacity and protect against any harmful chemicals or cell degeneration. A balanced and healthy diet can also help moderate body weight, especially when combined with daily exercise. Engaging in daily physical activities will not only help ensure a healthy body weight, but it can also help prevent early onset of Alzheimer's disease and dementia.

Exercise

In addition to eating healthy, getting regular exercise helps reduce the risk of dementia. In fact, engaging in regular physical activity can decrease your chances of developing Alzheimer's disease by fifty percent. Physical activity in this case does not mean running a few miles each day; even mild to moderate activity can help decrease the risk of developing this disease. Exercising 30 minutes a day, five days a week can help improve both brain and heart health. Some everyday activities that can contribute to this 30 minutes include swimming, walking, jogging, gardening, cleaning, walking up stairs, doing the laundry, and even grocery shopping. Essentially, any physical activity that works to increase your heart rate will help promote brain health. The reason for this connection between exercise and the decreased risk for Alzheimer's disease is believed to be due to the physical changes caused by exercise.

When an individual increases their heart rate through physical exercise, it causes their blood to pump through the body at a faster rate. This action in turn increases the number of small blood vessels that carry blood to the brain. With an increase in oxygen-rich blood being delivered to the brain, the brain is able to function at an increased capacity. In addition to forming small blood vessels, exercise can increase the number of connections between nerve cells. Nerve cell growth can also be attributed to increased exercise, particularly in the parts of the brain associated with learning and memory. When an individual begins developing Alzheimer's disease or dementia, many of the neural pathways in the brain become damaged or disappear entirely. Studies now show that regular physical exercise can help maintain these neural pathways, thus decreasing the risk for Alzheimer's disease and dementia, or at the very least slowing their progression considerably.

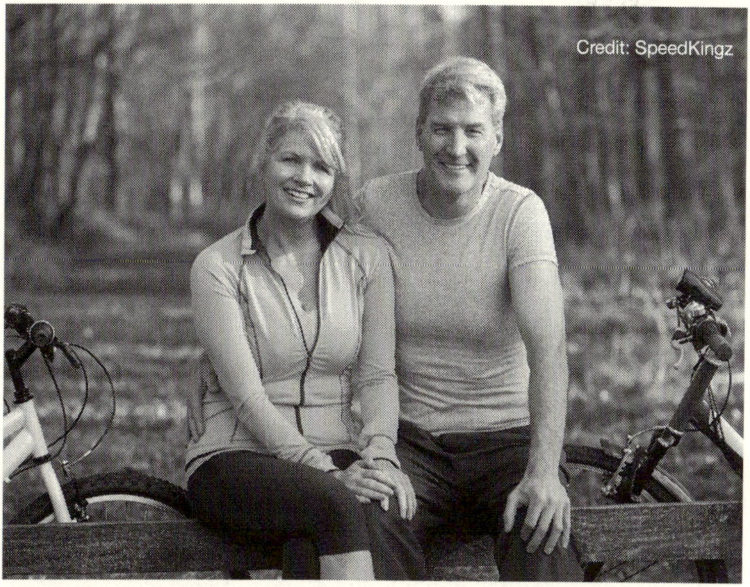

If you have a family history of Alzheimer's disease or dementia or have begun to show early signs of memory loss, exercise could be extremely beneficial. In a study of a group of individuals all genetically predisposed to Alzheimer's disease, those who did not exercise experienced brain shrinkage over the study's time period of a year and a half, whereas those who engaged in physical exercise did not. Scientists studied the area of the brain responsible for short-term and long-term memory, and the individuals who did not exercise experienced a shrinkage of approximately 3 percent over a year and a half in these areas. Those who participated in mild to moderate exercise showed no change to the memory centers of their brain. Similarly, recent studies indicate that strength or resistance training (e.g., weight lifting) can improve cognitive function in individuals with mild cognitive impairment, potentially even better than aerobic exercises.

Some people hear the word exercise and immediately think of running, jogging, or other activities that are not always enjoyed by the majority of people. However, exercise can be any physical activity that you enjoy doing that increases your heart rate. If you do not like running, or if it is physically painful for you, then consider another activity such as swimming, biking, walking, or skating. You are much more likely to stick with an exercise routine if you enjoy the activity. Similarly, it could be helpful to find a friend to exercise with, as this will encourage both of you to continue exercising. You and your friend, or group of friends, could plan to go to the gym a few times a week or plan to take a half hour walk each night. Setting up a regular schedule and including another person in your exercise routine can help make it more enjoyable. Creating goals can also increase your motivation. These goals should be attainable; if you set an unrealistic goal, then you will feel defeated when you do not succeed. Instead, begin with small, attainable goals, and be proud of yourself when you meet them. This success will then help you continue to meet larger exercise goals that you set as time goes on.

Typically, individuals who try to incorporate regular or daily exercise into their routines stop after a week or two, especially if they do not particularly enjoy exercising. If you can stick with an exercise routine for a month, the likelihood of it becoming a habit increases substantially. Creating a habit takes approximately 28 days, at which point the activity becomes routine. If you can commit to 30 minutes of moderate physical activity—such as walking or gardening—for 28 days, the activity will be much easier to continue, because it will become part of your daily routine. This exercise will then not only prove to be beneficial to your bodily health but to your brain health as well.

Although exercise in most forms is considered to be beneficial, high impact sports that have an increased risk of head injury—such as football, hockey, boxing, and rugby—can actually increase a person's risk for Alzheimer's disease and dementia. Repeated head injuries can cause damage to the brain, thus increasing the likelihood of cognitive impairment developing earlier in life. If you or a loved one are at risk for Alzheimer's disease or dementia and choose to begin exercising more regularly, make sure that there is not an increased risk of head injuries associated with that physical activity. Similarly, if you choose to exercise by riding a bike or roller skating, always make sure to wear a safety helmet in case of falls.

Beverages and Brain Health

When using nutrition to decrease your risk factors for developing dementia, many people overlook the importance of beverages. Coffee, tea, and red wine all have preventive qualities when it comes to memory loss. Tea and coffee both help memory and brain health due to their natural ingredients. Red wine, consumed in moderation, has been shown to benefit both heart and brain health. Adding these readily available drinks to your daily routine could prevent you or a loved one from developing Alzheimer's disease or dementia, delay the onset of the disease, or in many cases slow its progression in those who are already experiencing symptoms.

Coffee

Many individuals start their morning with a cup of coffee, or they have coffee at some point during the day. Research regarding the negative impacts of coffee has been circulating for years, but a significant amount of research is now being done regarding the connection between coffee consumption, improved memory, and lowering the risk factors for Alzheimer's disease, dementia, and general cognitive decline. Drinking three to five, six ounce cups of coffee per day can lead to improved memory retention and can significantly reduce your chances of developing Alzheimer's disease. In fact, for some individuals with Alzheimer's disease, coffee consumption can temporarily arrest the progression of the disease for a time, although the disease's progress cannot be halted indefinitely. If drinking caffeinated coffee, it is important to remember that the caffeine content can become detrimental to your health if too much is consumed. Six or more cups of coffee per day can begin to cause insomnia, restlessness, and gastrointestinal difficulties.

The reason why coffee can be beneficial is not entirely known, but many researchers have found that it is not due to the caffeine content alone. Caffeine does help people remember facts more effectively, but it is an ingredient in the coffee itself—both caffeinated and non-caffeinated—that ultimately proves beneficial to memory and brain structure.

Tea

Both black and green tea help delay the onset or slow progression of Alzheimer's disease and dementia. Black tea is thought to have this impact due to both the caffeine in the drink as well as the antioxidants in the tea leaves themselves. Similarly, drinking black tea improves memory, information processing, and learning. Generally, drinking one cup of black tea per day can produce these positive changes.

Green tea prevents some processes that could lead to the development of Alzheimer's disease or dementia. In fact, drinking green tea daily results in a 54% reduction in the risk of cognitive decline. The components of green tea reduce plaques that form in the brain; these plaques are thought to contribute to the cognitive decline associated with Alzheimer's disease. These plaques form and stick to parts of the brain associated with learning and memory. Eventually, they cause damage to that part of the brain. Researchers have found that green tea actually stops these plaques from forming by preventing them from sticking to healthy neurons in the brain. Additionally, the ingredients of the tea also lead to increased brain cell production and repairing of damaged neurons. These new and repaired cells lead to noticeable improvements in memory and learning within a short period of time.

If you or your loved one are at risk of developing Alzheimer's disease or dementia, or already have the disease, drinking one cup of green tea per day could be very beneficial. It is a small change, but it can lead to large improvements. Researchers also found that introducing more green tea did not have negative effects on the brain but rather showed a higher rate of improvement. Therefore, if you or a loved one want to drink two to three cups of green tea per day, it could be even more advantageous to brain health. However, more than five cups per day can cause negative side effects due to the caffeine content.

In addition to increasing memory, learning, and mental alertness, green tea consumption helps lower cholesterol levels. Drinking one cup of green tea per day for six months results in a decrease in total cholesterol as well as a marked decrease in "bad" cholesterol. As discussed in the decrease saturated fats and cholesterol section, high levels of cholesterol increase a person's risk for developing dementia. Therefore, a small change to you or your loved one's daily routine, such as drinking a cup of green tea, could have numerous beneficial effects.

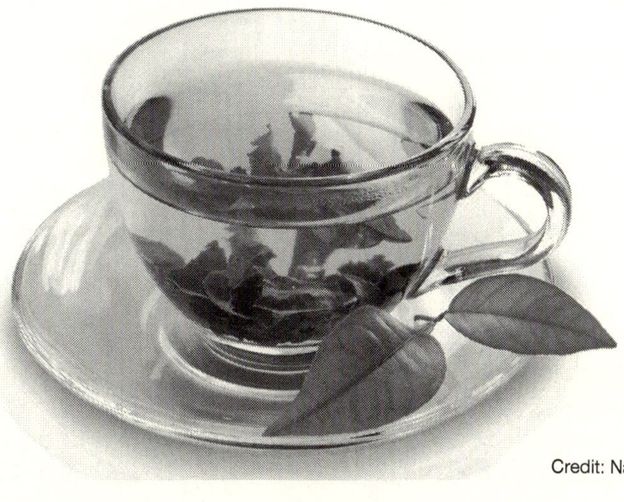

Credit: NataliTerr

Red wine

Similar to how green tea can lead to a decrease in plaque formation in the brain, an ingredient in red wine—an antioxidant called resveratrol—has almost the same effect. Drinking one glass of red wine per day could lead to a decrease in your risk for Alzheimer's disease or dementia. This is attributed to both the wine's ability to impact the formation of plaques as well as red wine's link to a decrease in cholesterol. This particular nutritional change should not be considered if you or your loved one have a history of alcohol abuse, liver problems, or are pregnant or breastfeeding. Additionally, while one glass of red wine a day can be beneficial, excessive alcohol consumption—four to five glasses a day or more—can actually lead to an increased risk of developing Alzheimer's disease or dementia.

Vitamin Deficiencies

Certain vitamins can be extremely important if you are trying to decrease your risk factors for Alzheimer's disease or dementia. The deficiency of some vitamins within the human body can cause adverse symptoms, including memory loss and difficulty connecting ideas. Many lifestyle and health factors can contribute to vitamin deficiencies due to vitamin absorption difficulties, including smoking, certain medications, low stomach acid content, antacids, Inflammatory Bowel Disease, and Crohn's disease. If vitamins, such as vitamin C and vitamin B_{12}, are deficient for too long, they can cause brain damage and put a person at increased risk for cognitive deficiencies—including both Alzheimer's disease

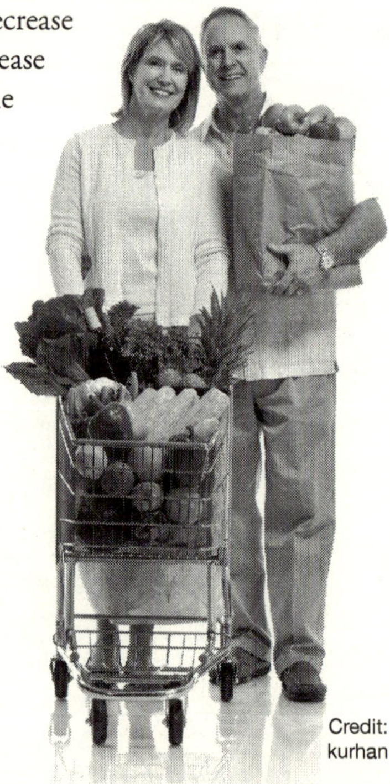

Credit: kurhan

and dementia. In addition, vitamin C and vitamin E, when consumed together, help reduce the risk of developing these disorders, or at least slow progression of the disease. In many cases, vitamin deficiencies are best treated by changing your diet to include foods high in those vitamins, but at times doctors will recommend that you begin taking a supplement in addition to dietary modifications.

Vitamin C

Vitamin C is exceptionally important in terms of brain health and cognitive development. Foods that are high in vitamin C not only help keep the immune system strong, they can also help improve memory performance. Many individuals who have Alzheimer's disease and dementia also have a vitamin C deficiency. While this vitamin deficiency alone will not cause the disease, it could help to speed progression and increase cognitive impairment. By working to increase your or your loved one's vitamin C intake, it could help slow the progression of the disease, and at the very least will contribute to your brain and body health in a positive manner. The checklist below highlights some foods that are high in vitamin C.

Checklist: Foods high in vitamin C

- Acidic fruits (oranges, lemons, limes, grapefruit, pineapple, kiwi, tomatoes)
- Berries (strawberries, raspberries, blackberries)
- Dark leafy greens (spinach, kale, salad greens)
- Green vegetables (broccoli, peas, okra)
- Cabbage family (cabbage, Brussels sprouts)
- Melons (cantaloupe, honey dew, papaya, mango, guava)
- Peppers (red bell, green bell, hot chili peppers)
- Other (cauliflower, winter squash, sweet potato)

Many supermarkets and health food stores sell vitamin C supplements, but incorporating foods high in vitamin C into your diet is really the best approach. These foods are absorbed more efficiently by the body, and they can provide other important vitamins and minerals that have a positive impact on brain health.

Additionally, taking too much supplemental vitamin C could lead to an excess amount of the vitamin in your body, which could result in negative side effects. It is much more difficult to consume dangerous levels of vitamin C through eating fruits and vegetables.

Vitamin B_{12}

Low levels of vitamin B_{12} can lead to an increased risk for Alzheimer's disease and dementia. This is likely due to the fact that B vitamins are important to neuron health and help maintain stable neuron pathways. When an individual develops Alzheimer's disease or dementia, their neural pathways begin to deteriorate, or shrink, causing less communication between neurons. This eventually results in cognitive decline. Therefore, a vitamin B_{12} deficiency at any point in your or your loved one's life could lead to decreased memory function and should be avoided.

Vitamin B_{12} deficiency is most common in older adults, vegetarians, and vegans. Vitamin B_{12} is found naturally in meat, seafood, and dairy sources, allowing most people to achieve healthy levels of the vitamin within their normal diets. However, if you or your loved one are a vegetarian or vegan—thus not eating meat or dairy products—it can limit the sources of vitamin B_{12} you consume on a daily basis. In these situations, you may need to take vitamin B_{12} supplements or consume sufficient amounts of non-meat or dairy foods that are high in the vitamin. Age can also be an important factor in vitamin B_{12} absorption, as it becomes more difficult for the body to absorb this vitamin after age 50. Absorption can also be compromised by some medical conditions, such as Crohn's disease, celiac disease, and reduced liver function. If you or a loved one have any medical conditions that reduce absorption of vitamin B_{12}, you should ensure that you are getting enough vitamin B_{12}, as this will decrease your risk of developing Alzheimer's disease or dementia. However, taking vitamin B_{12} supplements when you do not have a vitamin B_{12} deficiency does not improve memory or decrease your risk for Alzheimer's disease or dementia. Instead, you should aim to maintain healthy levels of vitamin B_{12} consumption, especially as you progress into your 50s and 60s.

Adults should consume 2.4 micrograms per day of vitamin B_{12}, a level that most people can maintain by eating a regular balanced diet. Women who are pregnant or breastfeeding will need to consume more each day to meet their body's needs. If you believe you are suffering from a vitamin B_{12} deficiency, or that you are not consuming enough vitamin B_{12} each day, check with your doctor before taking any supplements or changing your diet. Vitamin B_{12} levels can only be determined through a blood test.

Slowing the Progression of Alzheimer's Disease

Once your loved one is diagnosed with Alzheimer's disease, the progression could either move rapidly or slowly. Many factors have been shown to speed up the progression of this disease, including both stress and anxiety. Beyond that, however, it is commonly accepted that after diagnosis, individuals generally live between four and twenty years. Some individuals survive as long as twenty-five years after diagnosis. An area of research that has recently been getting a lot of attention is nutrition and Alzheimer's disease. Research has shown that certain dietary choices and nutritional habits can actually slow the progression of Alzheimer's disease for those who are in the mild to moderate stages. Changes that can be made include maintaining a healthy diet, eating foods that are considered to be brain healthy, and taking specific vitamins or eating vitamin-rich foods.

Balanced Diet

Eating a balanced diet is important for all individuals, not only those with Alzheimer's disease. However, this may be more important for your loved one with Alzheimer's disease, as poor nutrition can result in the worsening of Alzheimer's disease symptoms. A balanced diet contains a variety of foods including fruits, vegetables, grains, protein, and adequate fluids. Fruits and vegetables should make up approximately half of your loved one's daily nutritional intake. This can be in the form of fresh, frozen, or even canned fruits and vegetables. The other half of your loved one's diet should consists of grains and proteins, such as beans, fish, and high fiber fortified grains.

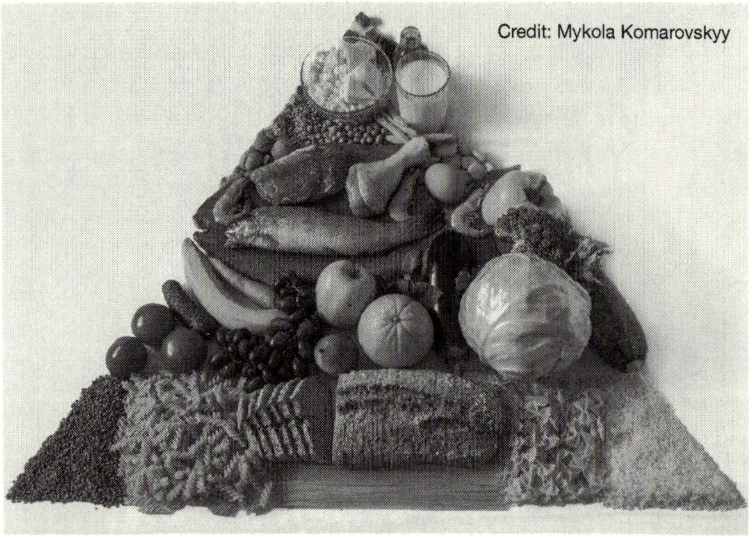

As Alzheimer's disease progresses, it can become more difficult for your loved one to maintain healthy eating habits due to decreased appetite, inability to recognize food, or difficulty swallowing. Below is a checklist highlighting some ways to help your loved one maintain his or her nutrition, even if these eating difficulties are present.

Checklist: Maintaining nutrition with eating and swallowing difficulties

- Serve bite-sized portions of foods that are easy to pick up and consume, which will also make chewing and swallowing easier.
- Grind foods, when possible, to make them easier to swallow.
- Serve soft, nutritious, foods such as applesauce, cottage cheese, canned fruits, and scrambled eggs.
- Prepare foods that have high nutritional value, but can be blended, including fruit or vegetable smoothies, pureed vegetables, and whipped potatoes.
- Avoid serving foods that could be difficult to chew completely, and/or that pose a choking risk. Some examples of this would be raw fruits or vegetables, which could instead be steamed, pureed, or both.

- Keep meals small and increase their frequency; for example, in place of three large meals a day, try five or six smaller meals throughout the day.
- Thicken liquids and soups to make them easier to swallow. This can be done by adding unflavored gelatin or food thickeners.
- If your loved one's sense of taste begins to be diminished, try to add natural sweeteners, such as honey, to food in order to make the food more appealing.
- Add strong spices to food to enhance its taste, but avoid adding too much salt as it can cause water retention and dehydration.
- Serve soft fruits and vegetables as snacks, such as bananas, peaches, oranges, and cooked vegetables.
- Prepare thickened soups and stews that contain large portions of vegetable, dairy, and grain products, as this will make it easier to get the most nutrition out of a single, easy to eat, meal.
- Serve soups and stews in a mug rather than a bowl so that your loved one does not have to struggle with using a spoon.

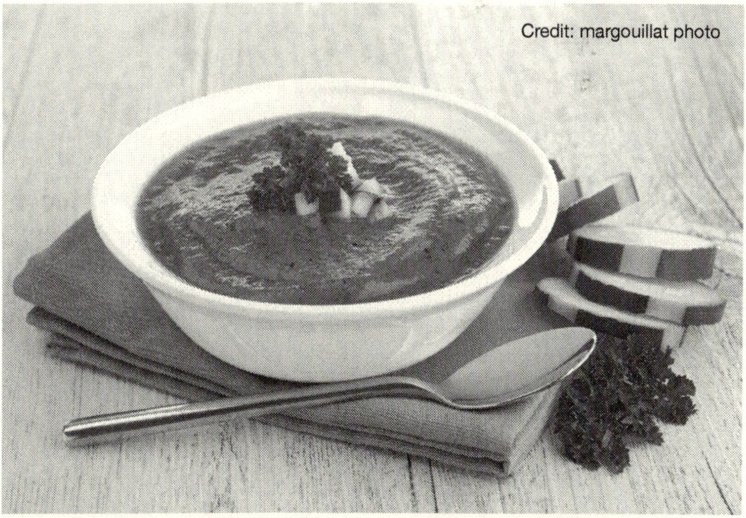

Credit: margouillat photo

- Serve foods that are liquid-based, as this can be very helpful in avoiding your loved one becoming dehydrated.

- Serve bite-sized pieces of melons, watermelon, and citrus fruits, as these fruits contain a lot of water, are nutritious, and are easy to chew.
- Prepare meats that are easy to chew, such as pulled pork, chop meat, or shredded chicken. Steak or thicker cuts of beef or chicken can become tough and difficult to chew and swallow, thus posing a choking risk.

Brain Healthy Foods

Several foods and food groups can help contribute to increased brain health. Often, this is due to the vitamins and antioxidants within the foods that protect brain cells and neural pathways in the brain. Many of these same foods have been proven to produce, or stimulate the production of, new neurons and pathways. These foods are often referred to as being "brain healthy." Some examples include green leafy vegetables as well as other dark fruits and vegetables. Foods high in omega 3 fatty acids, such as many types of fish, also promote brain health. These foods help decrease a person's risk factors for Alzheimer's disease and dementia, slow progression of the disease, and in some instances help improve memory function in the mild stage of disease. If you or your loved one are at risk for Alzheimer's disease or dementia, or are in the early stages of the disease, including these brain healthy foods into your diet could be beneficial.

Dark fruits and vegetables

Certain foods are more "brain healthy" or "protective" than others, and these can help your loved one's memory. These foods reduce damage to brain cells and in some instances increase memory retention and overall brain functioning. Many of these foods are dark-skinned fruits and vegetables, but in particular spinach, kale, and collard greens are shown to have the most potent and beneficial effects on brain cells. Dark leafy greens, such as spinach, have high amounts of carotenoids and flavonoids, which are nutrients that can help decrease mental decline by almost 40 percent. For the greatest impact, your loved one should eat three or more servings of these foods per day.

The main reason that many of these fruits and vegetables are considered to be brain healthy is because they contain high amounts of antioxidants. Antioxidants are most commonly found in fruits and vegetables and help prevent or delay cell damage. Some common forms of antioxidants found in brain healthy foods include vitamin C, vitamin E, and beta-carotene. All of these vitamins help delay the onset of Alzheimer's disease and dementia and/or help slow cognitive and physical decline in the earlier stages of the disease. The following checklist highlights fruits and vegetables that are rich in antioxidants and are onsidered to be brain healthy.

Checklist: Foods that are high in antioxidants

Vegetables:

- Spinach
- Kale
- Collard greens
- Brussel sprouts
- Broccoli
- Alfalfa sprouts
- Beets
- Corn
- Red peppers
- Eggplant

Credit: Robyn Mackenzie

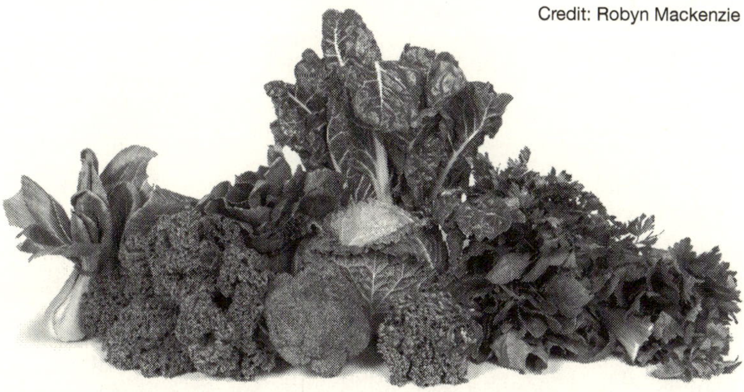

Fruits:

- Blueberries
- Raspberries
- Strawberries
- Blackberries
- Acai berries
- Elderberries
- Cranberries
- Prunes
- Raisins
- Plums
- Oranges
- Cherries

Omega 3 fatty acids help brain function

Omega 3 fatty acids can help lower your or your loved one's risk factors for Alzheimer's disease and dementia, and they can also help slow the progression of the disease in the early stages. Omega 3s can be found in several different types of foods, but they are mostly found in fish. The reason omega 3s can be so helpful to brain health is because they increase the number of neurons in the brain, produce protective chemicals in the brain, and reduce the formation of plaques and tangles. By consuming foods with this essential fatty acid, you can help improve your overall brain health and decrease cognitive decline.

Checklist: Foods that are high in omega 3

- Fresh tuna (this should be eaten no more than two times a month because it has a high mercury content)
- Salmon (wild is best)
- Mackerel
- Herring
- Sardines
- Trout
- Anchovy
- Sea bass

- Halibut
- Mussels
- Shrimp
- Oysters
- Grass-fed beef
- Krill oil and fish oil
- Flax seeds, or flax seed oil
- Canola oil
- Pumpkin seeds
- Mustard seeds
- Algae
- Walnuts
- Soybeans
- Tofu
- Brussels sprouts
- Cauliflower
- Green vegetables (both leafy and others)
- Edamame
- Fortified products (eggs, milk, cereal, etc.)
- Oatmeal

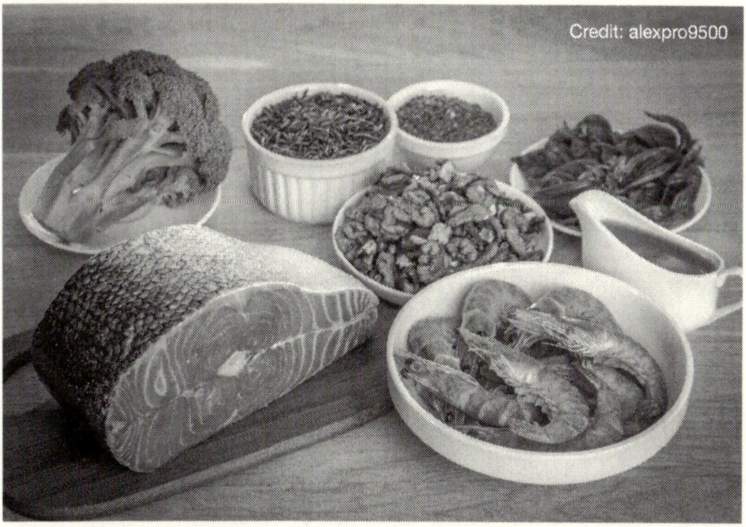

You'll notice that seafood, and especially fish, dominates the first half of this list. While eating fish is generally recognized as a healthy choice, mercury poisoning is considered to be a risk with certain varieties of fish. Specifically, king mackerel, marlin, orange roughy, shark, swordfish, tilefish, ahi tuna, and bigeye tuna are all fish that contain high levels of mercury; note that of these fish, only tuna and mackerel are on the checklist above. What does this mean? Potentially, if pregnant women are exposed to high levels of mercury, that could interfere with the brain development of their unborn children. Adults in general, however, have a low risk from mercury exposure. Cooking has no effect on the mercury levels in fish, and it isn't something you can taste, either. Other than mercury levels, PCBs and dioxins present another potential health hazard from eating fish.

The checklist below lays out some food safety facts to consider with regard to fish.

Checklist: Fish and shellfish safety guidelines

- Mercury exposure is primarily a risk for pregnant women, women who plan to become pregnant, women who are nursing, and children under the age of six, but most adults have low risk from mercury exposure.
- If an adult is concerned about exposure to mercury, that means limiting the consumption of fish high in mercury. *From Checklist: Foods that are high in omega 3*, that means limiting or avoiding the consumption of tuna and mackerel.
- Larger fish such as tuna and swordfish are likely to contain higher levels of mercury than smaller fish and shellfish such as squid, scallops, and sardines.
- Eat local, and in particular avoid fish imported from countries like China and Vietnam that have less rigorous management practices for ensuring harvested fish are safe. The US Food and Drug Administration only inspects about 2% of all fish imported to this country.
- Buy seafood from trusted sellers with high standards. Fresh fish is safe for purchase only if it is refrigerated or displayed on a bed of ice that is thick and fresh—that is, not melting. All fish should be well-separated in the display.

- Use your eyes, ears, and nose to select the best fish. Fish should be springy and resilient to the touch; it should not have an ammonia-like, fishy, or sour smell but should instead smell fresh and mild; and there should be no discoloration or darkening or drying around the edges.
- Any fish that will not be used within two days should be stored in a freezer.
- Thaw fish in the refrigerator overnight or, to thaw quickly, in a plastic bag immersed in cold water or in the microwave with the defrost setting, as long as the defrost cycle does not continue to the point that the fish is no longer icy and pliable.
- Cook most seafood to an internal temperature of 145°F.
- Seafood should never be left out of the refrigerator longer than two hours or one hour if the temperature is 90°F or above. For a picnic, pack seafood in ice. For parties, keep hot seafood hot and cold seafood cold.
- Throw away any shellfish with cracked or broken shells.
- Remember, higher levels of omega 3s are the potential benefit from eating many types of fish and shellfish. If you are concerned about the health risks of eating fish and shellfish or simply don't like seafood, then try the non-seafood items listed in *Checklist: Foods that are high in omega 3.*

If your loved one is in the early stages of Alzheimer's disease or dementia, adding foods rich in omega 3s could help improve memory and slow progression of the disease. These improvements are often seen quickly and can be long-lasting if omega 3 consumption and healthy dietary practices are consistently observed. Eating one to three servings of fish per week has the greatest positive benefits, especially when compared to taking fish oil supplements. Omega 3 supplements can be helpful, but your body will absorb and make use of the omega 3s present in natural sources more efficiently.

Although omega 3 fatty acids help improve memory and boost neuron development, the consumption of a consistently unhealthy and unbalanced diet can negate these positive benefits. For example, if you or your loved one eat three servings of healthy fish or other omega

3-rich foods a week but are otherwise eating foods high in saturated fat, cholesterol, and refined sugars, the omega 3 consumption will not prove beneficial. A healthy, balanced diet is essential to getting the most vitamins and minerals out of foods.

Positive benefits of omega 3 fatty acids have been seen in those with mild Alzheimer's disease and dementia; however, studies have shown that omega 3 consumption has not proved beneficial to those with moderate to severe Alzheimer's disease and dementia. It is best to start these nutritional changes before symptoms arise or at the first signs of cognitive decline. For individuals who carry the E4 allele, a genetic risk factor for Alzheimer's disease, omega 3s have not been shown to help slow progression of the disease or lessen symptoms, even in the earliest stages.

Mediterranean Diet

Individuals who live in the Mediterranean region have higher life expectancies than most populations and have a lower rate of individuals with dementia. For this reason, as well as other nutritional factors, the Mediterranean diet is recommended as one way to help lower your risk for dementia. This particular dietary approach can also have a positive effect on those in the early stages of dementia, helping to noticeably slow progression of the symptoms. Additionally, the Mediterranean diet decreases the risk for heart disease and stroke.

The main component of this dietary approach is eating large portions of fruits, vegetables, whole grains, and legumes. Most, if not all, meals should be made up of these ingredients, with approximately six or more servings of fruits and vegetables per day. In addition, whole grains are very important and should be included in most meals. Fish and seafood are another essential component of this diet, providing protein and omega 3s. Most who follow the Mediterranean diet consume fish or seafood at least twice a week, if not more frequently. Conversely, red meat should be eaten infrequently, no more than once or twice per month. Poultry, such as chicken and turkey, can be eaten in place of red meat.

In addition to limiting consumption of red meat, the Mediterranean diet also suggests avoiding butter, salt, high fat dairy products, and refined sugars. Butter can be easily replaced in most cases by olive oil, which is a large component of this diet. Extra virgin and virgin olive oil are the healthiest types to use, as they contain rich antioxidants. In place of salt, other herbs and spices can be used to add flavor to food as well as to provide additional nutritional benefits. For example, the spice turmeric, often used in curries, helps prevent the formation of plaques in the brain, which could contribute to the development of Alzheimer's disease. High fat dairy products can easily be replaced by skim or fat free options.

Nuts, seeds, and red wine are also among the suggested components of the Mediterranean diet. Nuts and seeds are high in both fiber and protein, helping to keep a person full for longer and contributing to a balanced diet. Approximately one handful of nuts per day is recommended, and you should avoid nuts that have been heavily salted or roasted. Some suggestions include walnuts, pistachios, peanuts, almonds, and cashews. Red wine, in moderation, is also recommended a few times a week. See the red wine section for more information on this beverage.

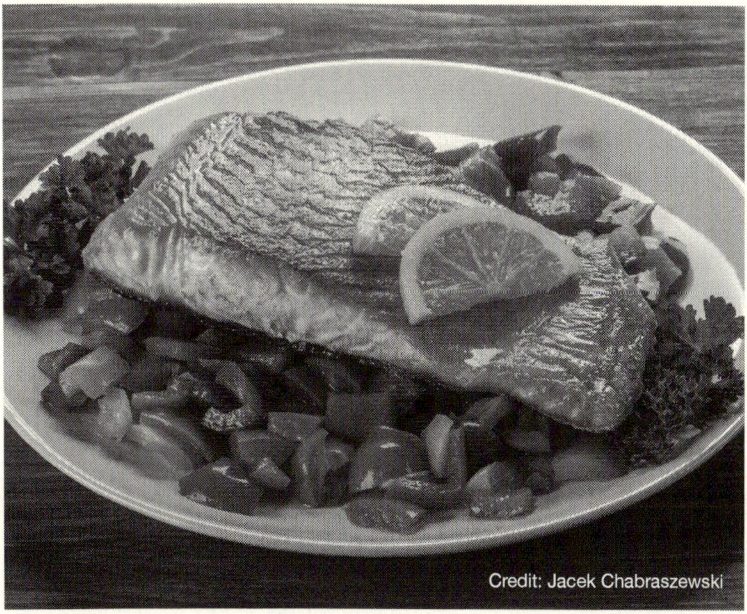

Credit: Jacek Chabraszewski

Conclusion

Alzheimer's disease and dementia are often very difficult diseases to confront, both for those who have the ailment and their loved ones. As more research is conducted on these diseases, helpful information is released to the public. Research on nutritional changes is a growing and increasingly popular field, especially as more data is collected regarding the many positive benefits of a healthy diet. Whether you have a family history of Alzheimer's disease or dementia, are at risk for the disease, or have a loved one who is suffering, the nutritional changes discussed here could be very helpful. Many of these dietary modifications decrease a person's risk factors for developing Alzheimer's disease or dementia or slow progression of the disease. In addition, most of the health guidelines discussed in this book not only benefit brain health but overall health as well.

About the Authors

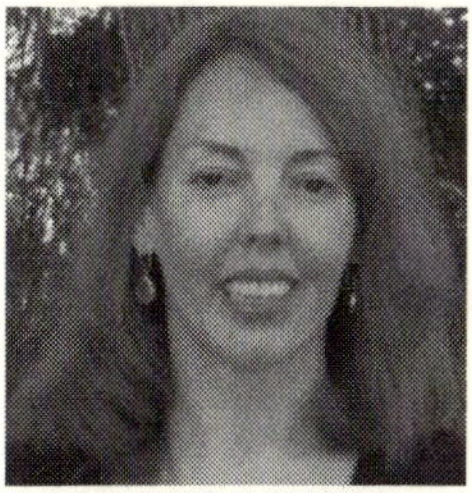

Laura Town

Laura Town has authored numerous publications of special interest to the aging population. She has expertise in the field of finance as a co-author on Finance: Foundations of Financial Institutions and Management published by John Wiley and Sons, and she has contributed to several online nursing courses and texts. She has also written for the American Medical Writers Association, and her work has been published by the American Society of Journalists and Authors. As an editor, Laura has worked with Pearson Education, Prentice Hall, McGraw-Hill Higher Education, John Wiley and Sons, and the University of Pennsylvania to create both on-ground and online courses and texts. She is currently the President-Elect of the Indiana chapter of the American Medical Writers Association.

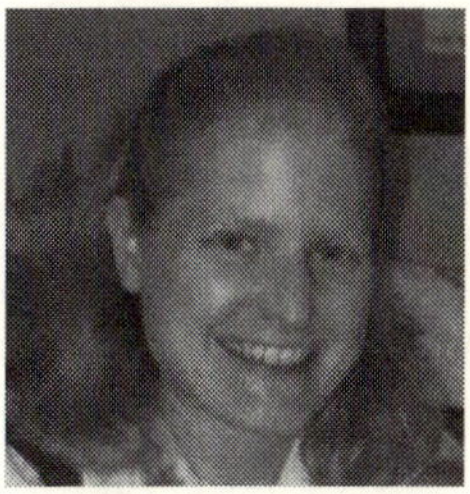

Karen Kassel

Karen Kassel received her Ph.D. in Pharmacology from the Department of Pharmacology and Experimental Neurosciences at the University of Nebraska Medical Center in Omaha, NE, where she was the recipient of an American Heart Association fellowship and several regional and national awards for her research on G protein-coupled receptor signaling in airways. She then pursued post-doctoral research projects at the University of North Carolina-Chapel Hill and the University of Kansas Medical Center, again receiving fellowships from the PhRMA Foundation and the American Heart Association, respectively. She has published research in the American Journal of Pathology, Journal of Biological Chemistry, and Journal of Pharmacology and Experimental Therapeutics. In 2012, Karen joined the editorial staff at WilliamsTown Communications, an editing firm that specializes in educational products for undergraduate- and graduate-level students. At WTC, Karen specializes in producing educational products related to the sciences and healthcare. In addition, Karen is board-certified for editing life sciences (BELS-certified).

A Note from the Authors

Thank you for purchasing our book! If you have any questions for us, feel free to reach out to the authors via twitter: @laurawtown, @KarenKassel1. We would appreciate it if you would take the time to review our book on Amazon, as our book's visibility on Amazon depends on reviews.

Worldwide, over forty million people suffer from Alzheimer's disease, and that number is expected to increase significantly within the next fifteen years. In the United States, five million people have the disease, and that is expected to triple by the year 2050.

Despite these large numbers, you may feel alone. I (Laura) know that when I started caring for my father, who had early-onset Alzheimer's disease, I felt alone. Although my father has passed away, I am haunted by what he suffered and how difficult it was to care for him. However, now I know that there are people, resources, and organizations that can help others going through this same struggle.

One major concern of caregivers is knowing how to provide adequate nutrition for their loved one. We hope that the information in the *Alzheimer's Roadmap* series will ease some of your stress. The information provided in this book not only provides guidelines on what types of foods will most benefit your loved one's cognitive function but also how to prepare those foods so your loved one can consume them easily and safely. In addition, we have included resources at the end of this book to provide additional information to help you through this process.

More Titles from Laura Town and Karen Kassel

Alzheimer's Roadmap **series:**

Long-Term Care Insurance, Power of Attorney, Wealth Management, and Other First Steps

Dementia, Alzheimer's Disease Stages, Treatment Options, and Other Medical Considerations

Advance Directives, Durable Power of Attorney, Wills, and Other Legal Considerations

Paying for Healthcare and Other Financial Considerations

Home Safety Checklist Guide and Caregiver Resources for Medication Safety, Driving, and Wandering

Home Care, Long-term Care, Memory Care Units, and Other Living Arrangements

*Caregiver Resources: From Independence to a Memory Care Unit**

Caregiver Resources for Helping with Activities of Daily Living

*This is a combination of the home safety and living arrangements books.

Resources

Alzheimer's Association
225 N. Michigan Ave., Fl. 17
Chicago, IL 60601-7633
Phone: 800-272-3900
Fax: 866-699-1246
Email: info@alz.org
Website: http://www.alz.org

Alzheimer's Foundation of America
322 Eighth Ave., 7th fl.
New York, NY 10001
Phone: 866-232-8484
Fax: 646-638-1546
Website: www.alzfdn.org

Choose MyPlate
Website: http://choosemyplate.gov/supertracker-tools/daily-food-plans.html
Choose MyPlate is a good resource for creating a customized daily food plan.

Alzheimer's Roadmap series
Purchase on Amazon:

Long-Term Care Insurance, Power of Attorney, Wealth Management, and Other First Steps

Dementia, Alzheimer's Disease Stages, Treatment Options, and Other Medical Considerations

Advance Directives, Durable Power of Attorney, Wills, and Other Legal Considerations

Paying for Healthcare and Other Financial Considerations

Home Safety Checklist Guide and Caregiver Resources for Medication Safety, Driving, and Wandering

Home Care, Long-term Care, Memory Care Units, and Other Living Arrangements

*Caregiver Resources: From Independence to a Memory Care Unit**

Caregiver Resources for Helping with Activities of Daily Living

*This is a combination of the home safety and living arrangements books.

Reference List

Adams, N. (2013). Benefits of juicing vs. eating your vegetables. *Livestrong*. Retrieved from http://www.livestrong.com/article/251138-benefits-of-juicing-vs-eating-your-vegetables/

Alzheimer's Association. (2016). Retrieved from http://www.alz.org/

Alzheimer's Drug Discovery Foundation. (2014). Retrieved from http://www.alzdiscovery.org/

Alzheimer's Society. (2013). Eating and drinking. Retrieved from http://www.alzheimers.org.uk/site/scripts/documents_info.php?documentID=149

American Heart Association. (2016). Saturated Fats. Retrieved from http://www.heart.org/HEARTORG/GettingHealthy/NutritionCenter/HealthyEating/Saturated-Fats_UCM_301110_Article.jsp

Cleveland Clinic. (2014). Nutrition for Alzheimer's disease. Retrieved from http://my.clevelandclinic.org/health/diseases_conditions/hic_Alzheimers_and_Dementia_Overview/hic_Exercise_and_Alzheimers_Disease/hic_Nutrition_for_Alzheimers_Disease

Davis, J. C., Bryan, S., Marra, C. A., Sharma, D., Chan, A., Beattie, B. L., Graf, P., & Liu-Amrose, T. (2013). An economic evaluation of resistance training and aerobic training versus balance and toning exercises in older adults with mild cognitive impairment. PLoS One, 8(5), e63031.

Downey, M. (2014, August). How green tea protects against Alzheimer's disease. *Life Extension Magazine.* Retrieved from http://www.lef.org/Magazine/2014/8/How-Green-Tea-Protects-Against-Alzheimers-Disease/Page-01

Food and Drug Administration. (2015). Buy, store & serve safe food. Retrieved from http://www.fda.gov/Food/FoodborneIllnessContaminants/BuyStoreServeSafeFood/ucm077331.htm.

Food for the Brain. Action plan for dementia & Alzheimer's. (2012). Retrieved from http://www.foodforthebrain.org/nutrition-solutions/dementia-and-alzheimer%E2%80%99s-disease/action-plan-for-dementia-alzheimer%E2%80%99s.aspx

Haiken, M. (2013, June 30). Green tea may prevent Alzheimer's disease, says four new studies. *Forbes*. Retrieved from http://www.forbes.com/sites/melaniehaiken/2013/06/30/green-tea-may-prevent-alzheimers-say-four-new-studies/

Harvard School of Public Health. (2016). Fish: Friend or foe? Retrieved from http://www.hsph.harvard.edu/nutritionsource/fish/.

Hu, N., Yu, J., Wang, Y., Sun, L., & Tan, L. (2013). Nutrition and the risk of Alzheimer's disease. *BioMed Research International*, 2013 (5248204), 1-12.

Jicha, G., & Swaminathan, A. (2014). Nutrition and prevention of Alzheimer's dementia. *Frontiers in Aging Neuroscience*, 6(282), 1-25.

Mayo Clinic. (2016). Retrieved from http://www.mayoclinic.org/

MedlinePlus. (2016). Retrieved from http://www.nlm.nih.gov/medlineplus/

National Resources Defense Council. (2016). Mercury guide. Retrieved from https://www.nrdc.org/stories/mercury-guide.

National Resources Defense Council. (2015). The smart seafood buying guide. Retrieved from https://www.nrdc.org/stories/smart-seafood-buying-guide.

Reynolds, G. (2014, July 2). Can exercise reduce Alzheimer's risk? *The New York Times*. Retrieved from http://well.blogs.nytimes.com/2014/07/02/can-exercise-reduce-alzheimers-risk/?_r=0

Sifferlin, A. (2012, July 16). Mind your reps: Exercise, especially weight lifting, helps keep the brain sharp. *Time*. Retrieved from http://healthland.time.com/2012/07/16/mind-those-reps-exercise-especially-weight-lifting-helps-keep-your-brain-sharp/

Smith, M., Robinson, L., & Segal, J. (2016). Alzheimer's and dementia prevention: How to reduce your risk and protect your brain as you age. Retrieved from http://www.helpguide.org/articles/alzheimers-dementia/alzheimers-and-dementia-prevention.htm

Additional Titles from Omega Press

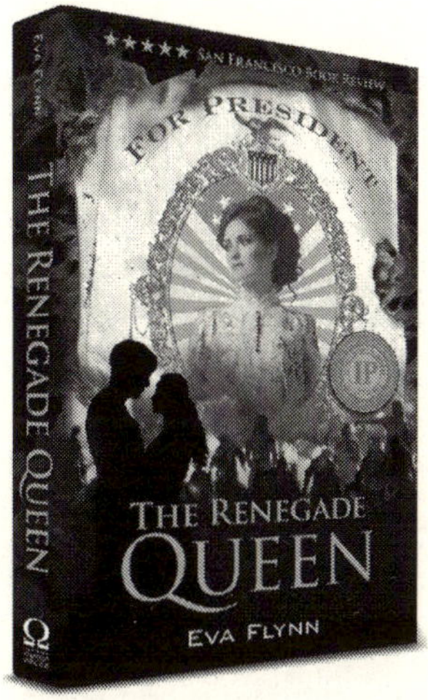

Available on Amazon.com

Born into poverty, sold into marriage, and nominated for President before women had the right to vote, Victoria Woodhull was nearly erased from history.

Discover the forgotten true story of this amazing woman, who overcame an abusive childhood, a coercive marriage, and the scorn of her society to fight for equality in life and love.

"Flynn hews closely to historical facts as she tells the story of Victoria Woodhull, a suffragist and reformer who worked as a fraudulent clairvoyant, opened a Wall Street brokerage with her sister, spent time in jail on obscenity charges, and ran for president in 1872. Flynn turns a history with no shortage of drama into compelling fiction, with a vivid setting and strong secondary characters, particularly Victoria's unfiltered younger sister and frequent sidekick, Tennessee. ...The woman known to the tabloids of her era as 'Mrs. Satan' is rendered as both driven and flawed, a fully realized character who will keep readers turning the pages."

—Kirkus

"This amazingly good debut novel by Eva Flynn stars Victoria Woodhull, a figure so outrageous and improbable that most of Flynn's readers will be tempted at first to think she's an invention of the author. And yet, no! ... Flynn embarks on the story of this remarkable woman with unabashed enthusiasm, giving us her upbringing, her loves, her controversies, and the controversies that attended this figure Flynn calls a 'forgotten feminist.' Flynn's storytelling is so energetic and her characters so vividly drawn that in addition to being eye-opening on many levels ..., it is also a page-turner."

—Historical Novel Society

Made in the USA
Middletown, DE
06 February 2020

84281768R00026